INTUITIVE MEDICINE

Also by Vera Dragilyova

IDEASTHESIA

CURVES IN CULTURE

THE UNKNOWN UNKNOWNS

FOOD FORMULAS

INTUITIVE MEDICINE

Zany Cures for the Incurable

Vera Dragilyova

Verarta Books

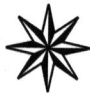

CONTENTS

INTRODUCTION

This book is a companion to Ideasthesia, which is the first book of its kind on the topic of Ideasthesia in the world. Ideasthesia is a rare neuropsychological phenomenon that augments human thinking, where abstract thought is processed in physical terms, in any of the five senses, allowing for a much more concrete and comprehensive analysis of otherwise abstruse material. The author shares the insight that her idesthetic visualizations have provided about human disease, its causes, and cures.

Many diseases are still considered incurable. However, the author suggests that, in her mental modeling, virtually all of them do have a specific cause. The motto of the book is: What if?

Modern medical science is prejudiced against the unknown, or is in complete denial of it, at least, the way it is practiced and experienced in an average doctor's office. Medicine is conservative because it is very risk-averse. It says that what it does not know— does not exist, and so doctors overlook many signs and symptoms, because they have been instructed to do so. Meanwhile, they could have been collecting and reporting valuable data to medical research institutions,—if only official science would open itself to the unknown and have it built into the research process, from the grassroots.

If the ideas in this book seem zany, it is only an indicator that they are veering away from the status quo, and it is there that their merit lies. Do not reject zaniness based on what you know, but give it a chance, based on what you don't. Zany ideas might be wrong, but the ideas they inspire might be right.

Disclaimer.

This book is a compilation of ideas for educational purposes only, and is not meant to diagnose or treat any disease. Its sole purpose is to stimulate discussion on medical topics, offering alternative views, which are nothing more than hypotheses.

MY STORY

Before you decide that my book is an encyclopedia of insanity and nonsense, let me tell you my story and explain how I came up with all the zany ideas that the title of this promises to offer.

It all started when I was just a few years old. I had an encyclopedia of medicine on a bookshelf, right next to my bed. Curiosity wouldn't have it any other way: the minute I started with the first random page in the middle of the book, I was hooked forever. The most fascinating idea was that there was human disease at all! But why? Why is there disease? Disease felt like a negative space, where the damage is done by something invisible, with only the results evident, but not the cause. It is like a hurricane that crushes buildings, but one cannot see the air that it is made of. I knew right away that there was an agent behind all this destruction of human body.

My grandmother spent most of her life in an experimental epidemiology lab, working on a miracle medicine that would strengthen the human immune system, to where it would become impenetrable to any known disease. It was during the Soviet Union era, and my father told me that, once she discovered something that met the standards, her project was suddenly sealed. No one will ever know, but the mystery has lingered and gnawed at me from the inside, like a parasite, all my life.

My other grandmother has been a natural healer for as long as I can remember, and I read all her books, neatly tucked onto a little shelf near her armchair. I would sit for hours and just read them like a detective story, unable to unglue my eyes or mind from the pages. We barely ever went to see a doctor: there was always my grandma to treat us with her herbs. I got used to the bitter taste of herbs, early in life, and it never bothered me to drink tea without any sugar ever since.

Bitterness, however, was not the worst of the tastes I had to withstand in the name of good health:

4

my grandma also gave me a concoction of milk, baking soda, butter, alcohol, and some other secret ingredients that felt explosive to my brain. A lethal, overwhelming, mind-blasting mixture, if you ask me! If I could drink that, I could do anything in life. It felt worse than being stung by fire ants in the coming of age ritual in the Amazon—or at least, that is what I imagine. Sometimes, my grandma gave me a straight shot of vodka. That was actually easier to withstand! And until now, I absolutely cannot stand alcohol. It reminds me of being sick and tortured, and I am physically and mentally allergic to it.

As I continued to read and re-read the medical encyclopedias, I started getting more and more intense visions of what was happening in each disease. For years, I thought that everyone else thought the same way, but finally, I discovered that my brain did work differently. What I have is called Ideasthesia. This is when the brain projects abstract thinking into visual, tactile, and other sensory channels, to where the thinker can see and mentally touch their thoughts. Yes, it sounds strange, but I don't know how to describe it better. Since we cannot see diseases, or their causes, or pathogens, or any of the processes involved,—thinking about them is abstract. None of it can be touched, picked up, taken apart, and studies, unless it is in the mind of an Ideasthete like me. In my mind, all those processes are physically manifested, and I can do with them what I can usually do with common physical objects in everyday reality.

The question is: does the insight I get in my mental world have any merit or significance to fighting actual diseases that actual people get? Well, for years, I had no idea, and entertained my visions, nonetheless. About twenty years ago, I read a medical article, published by Harvard University. It talked about a hypothesis that cancer was caused by a virus, and the light lit inside my head. It was rather like an explosion!

"Yes, exactly!"—I thought to myself,—"I knew it all along, I actually saw it in my head, all this time!" At the time, that was a groundbreaking scientific news. Before that moment, I never even dared speaking of my mental visions, and least of all, in the sciences. However, from that moment on, I knew that there was something to all this phantasmagoric world that lived inside me.

At the same time, I continued to treat myself with the treatments that my grandma taught me, and coming up with new ones, as new things happened to my body. I was never really sick, but little things needed to be treated. For example, my knees started hurting when I lived in San Diego. I went to see a doctor, two doctors, actually, and they both said that there was nothing wrong with me. One of them said that it might be that my bones were malformed! Hm, that was not something I just accepted as the ultimate verdict, and tried drinking apple cider vinegar with water every day instead. I did it because I kept visualizing that the cause of knee pain and swelling was some kind of a pathogen. I could see it 3D in my knees, like some kind of a cloud of little luminescent particles. I envisioned that apple cider vinegar, like many other anti-bacterial, anti-viral, anti-fungal, and generally anti-pathogen remedies would somehow render my body an unfriendly chemical environment, so that the pathogen would either die, or fall asleep, or leave.

Well, the pain went away in mere two days! The knee problem happened to my mother and my father, and my sister. They all got better from taking apple cider vinegar. All of them. A friend had COPD (poorly functioning lungs), and no medical treatment worked, so I told him to take vinegar, too. Guess what? He got better rather quickly, and then swore by it, from then on walking around with a cup of vinegar solution in his hand. This is just one tiny speck in the sea of cases that worked, based on my mental modeling of diseases and the results that this modeling provided to me.

I now live by these visualizations. Almost everything I read now, in any field, turns out to be only a confirmation of what I already know, and that gives me confidence in thinking that, at least, I might be on the right track with my visualizations.

Over the years, I have compiled my observations into a notebook, and from there this tiny book was born. It certainly does not cover everything there is to cover, but only offers some fundamental ideas that might help finding cures for the incurable diseases of modern times—and safe precious human lives.

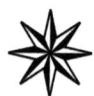

CAUSES OF DISEASE

What does it mean "to catch a cold"? Do you reach out and grab it, or do you let it land on the palm of your hand, just like a snowflake? No, none of it. You don't actually catch a cold, you either get invaded by new bacteria that start a colony inside you, or you let your old resident bacteria overbreed inside you, taking advantage of the low temperature, or of your temporary weakness. There is nothing romantic about it: it is all about pathogens. It feels something like hearing that Santa Claus does not really exist!

In fact, humans are walking and talking bacteria. We are parasites, living off of the earth, coexisting with it, and it has not been able to kill us off, all this time. Yet, we are not alone. It is a war of the worlds! Invisible to us, there are billions of organisms just like us, living alongside us, and inside us, and we don't even know it. In fact, our body contains pounds of bad and good bacteria. We sleep, eat, dream about the future, while they are viciously chewing our flesh.

And, we would never know they were there, if we didn't get sick once in a while, and asked ourselves: who is the culprit to be punished for all this? The causes of a disease are not so simple: they consist of a whole chain of events, and always involve a whole complex of factors that must come together, in order for us to get sick.

Who done it?

We have to be weak enough to be susceptible to disease, but how weak does it have to be? A lack of vitamins prevents our bodies from building its defenses, simply because they run out of raw materials. You can't build a brick house without the bricks, no matter how much you try to make other materials resemble it. Toxins further destroy our tissues, tearing down the last walls of defense we have our bodies against disease. We get toxins from the air we breathe and the food we eat, as well as producing toxins ourselves, when under stress. Finally, we are weakened. But is that all that is needed for disease? What is disease? It is not merely a malfunction of our bodies. That alone would not make us nearly as sick as we are. Where does the cause start, at which point? One could go as far as saying that the reason we die is because we are born.

For many years, I have been modeling in my mind the many factors of human disease: genetics, environment, the many symptoms, history of onset, the rate of spread, rates of recovery. Over and over again, I have arrived at the conclusion that the most culpable factor is pathogens, but only in combination with lack of vitamins, toxins and stress.

To my great terror, I have discovered that it is majority of diseases, especially the ones we consider incurable, are caused by pathogens that take advantage of our malaise and invade us. Our weakness coupled with pathogens is what causes the disease. Pathogens on their own are powerless against us, if our immune system is strong and can prevent them from penetrating our body. So, if a healthy individual comes across a pathogen, no disease will sprout. If a weak person does not meet a pathogen—no great disease will take place either. All genetic, physical, and psychosomatic causes combined do not amount to justify even the tiniest fraction of the totality of human disease. It is in the meeting of the two that the whole world finds its onus of suffering, from the beginning of time.

Health formula.

There are many ways of looking at causes of disease. One could construct a formula out of the four main factors that influence health, which is the opposite of disease:

Health=Vitamins—Pathogens—Toxins—Stress

Here, health is synonymous with immune system, where vitamins make it stronger, and pathogens, toxins, and stress—make it weaker. Pathogens are viruses, bacteria, fungi, parasites, and virulent proteins, like prions that cause Mad Cow disease.

What makes pathogens attack us?

Pathogens are everywhere, including inside us, but the two main determinants of whether they will attack us are how strong we are and their sheer number. There is a concept of quorum sensing in the world of microorganisms, among all pathogens, according to my modeling. They communicate with each other to decide whether they are strong enough in number to attack the host, each having its own communication system. Their strength is determined by estimating how weak we are relative to how many of them it would be necessary to succeed in their attack.

A weak immune system sends out chemical signals to pathogens, inviting them to feast, just like a few crumbs of bread on the ground will soon gather a whole flock of birds, appearing from nowhere. Pathogens read our body like a code, in order to decide when and whether they should attack. Two of the main invitation signals are high acidity and inflammation, but there are others, such as presence of heavy metals and free radicals.

Bacteria produce acidic waste products, as they devoir our tissues, and higher acidity than would be normal for a particular tissue signals to viruses and other pathogens that it is a good time and place to invade. It is not merely about the pH level, it also has to do with a particular chemical makeup of the acid that bacteria smell from far away: typical crowd-thinking. Viruses, in particular, are like vultures: if someone is already feasting on something, they will be there soon, to avoid wasting their effort in attacking something that is healthy and impenetrable. It is because viruses have to penetrate cell walls, in order to deposit their genetic material, and make the cell start producing copies of them, instead of what the body of the host usually produces. It is similar to the principle of cancer, and guess what? Cancer is number one disease that is absolutely contagious and is absolutely caused by a pathogen. Which one? I don't know. That is for medical researchers to establish. All I know is that it acts exactly like a vicious invasive mushroom-slash-virus, invading the host cells. More about cancer—later. So, yes, it is the feces of bacteria that are acidic, and when other pathogens detect them, they come over and take over. Our cells, whose walls are weakened by bacteria, are unable to fight off viruses and other pathogens, and it is an easy catch, once bacteria have settled in.

Inflammation.

Inflammation is a bodily reaction to a bacterial invasion, as well as to the damage done by toxins that both come from the environment, via air and food, but also produced internally from stress. We chemically interact with our environment. Our skin absorbs toxins from the surfaces we touch, and even from the objects with which we have no direct contact. Everything emanates their constituents into the air, which we then breath in, and then even our skin absorbs them.

Inflammation can also be caused by an autoimmune reaction of the body fighting off a pathogen, or by physical repeated abuse of a particular tissue. Smokers chronically abuse their lung and other tissues, and that is how cancer is invited to attack them. People in polluted cities suffer from all kinds of inflammation, and so invite pathogens in. Food that is poisoned by pesticides, GMO, and other harmful additives and manipulations, also acts as an irritant, causing long-term inflammation, which in turn is a beacon of hope for all the pathogens that make humans sick.

It is quite disgusting, when you zoom in and see the picture! If you could only see all the tools of torture these creatures use against us, and how they massacre our tissues—you would not just vomit, you might need PTSD treatment. So, wisely, nature protects us by not endowing us with microscopic vision. Otherwise, we would go insane.

Disease is a story.

Where exactly does a disease start? Does it start with our weakening, with stress from getting stuck in traffic, with breathing in second-hand smoke, or from having too little acid in our stomach to kill off the incoming bacteria? Or does it start with being exposed to a pathogen and catching a disease? Disease does not start at the point of the first symptom, but it starts with our birth, where our genetic material is already predisposed to be either vulnerable or not to certain diseases. Then, our environment has to be just right for the genetic material we have, and then, the right pathogen has to be introduced to us, just at the time when we are weak and unable to fight it off. So, catching a disease is not that easy, considering that evolution has culled off most of the genes that make us susceptible, and considering that it takes many circumstances to come together just right, for a particular disease to start. The problem is that there are a myriad diseases, caused by a myriad of pathogens, with a myriad of predisposing genetic and environmental characteristics. With so much statistical variety, we are bound to get one disease or another.

Yet, even at the moment, when all stars are in the right position, and it is a golden hour for a pernicious pathogen, as it sets its eyes on us, the target, there is still a story to be told. Each disease is an unpredictable process, a battle between the good and evil, where we are good, and pathogens are evil —we like to think that. In the end, either the disease or the host will win. We don't usually start telling the story until a penetration by a pathogen happens, and a binding between a pathogen and a human. Then, struggle ensues. This is the point where we might find out that we are sick. Or we might not even be aware of it. Our body can also be silently fighting many diseases, without even letting us know, while we are going about our usual business, completely asymptomatic. However, fighting any disease does tax our adrenal glands, and is experienced as stress by our body, which can eventually manifest itself as loss of energy, growing superficial belly and visceral fat, acne, dull skin tone, thyroid function imbalances, general weight gain or loss, swelling, edema, and all kinds of other "strange" symptoms that don't seem to point to any kind of a particular disease.

If the disease is fought off quietly, we start feeling more energetic and live on. If our immune system is unable to overpower the pathogen, it will enter a critical stage that will be brought into our awareness. Curiously, all diseases go through this story arch: hook, development, climax, and resolution. Anyone who has survived malaria or any type of a tropical fever will clearly recognize this trajectory, because in those diseases, it is particularly pronounced.

Swelling and edema.

Swelling and edema merit particular mention, because, according to my modeling, they are one of the most common symptoms of fighting a disease, or, at least, dealing with a high content of toxins in the body. Swelling can be caused by air, fluids, or expanding tissues, but edema is usually caused by an increased amount of water content. Swelling is a sign of inflammation, and edema has a specific function, as I can see it. Edema seems to be a body mechanism that changes the ratio of toxins to water in a solution, therefore, making toxins less damaging to the body. At a lower concentration, toxins lose their potency and cannot do as much harm, as they could at higher concentrations. It is like with herbal tinctures—the higher concentration of herb, the more potent the tincture overall. It is the same with poisons: the higher concentration—the more noxious they are. A similar process takes place with common salt: the more salt we eat, the more water our body retains, in order to keep the amount of salt low, relative to the amount of fluid that surrounds it.

Finally, edema becomes exaggerated, when in addition to toxins, the body is fighting pathogens that produce waste materials, poisonous to the body. During natural detoxification, the body retains more water, as a reservoir and a medium for transportation of poison out of the tissues. As soon as toxins and pathogens are ushered out into liver, kidneys, and other detoxifying organs, and out of the body, the extra water is eliminated.

It is not genetic, it is contagious.

They say that some diseases are genetic because they tend to run in families, and are absolutely not contagious. Like diabetes, for example. However, it may be that they are contagious, but need a repeated close contact of people to precipitate their numbers and quorum sensing confidence to attack, which is conveniently available in families living together. I wonder what the studies of relatives living separately would show, as compared to those living in close proximity, all things being equal.

It is not auto-immune, it is contagious.

They also say that auto-immune diseases are not contagious, because it is your own body fighting itself, and no one can catch a body behavior. That is the mental model that is universal in modern medicine.

However, according to my modeling, virtually all auto-immune disease are contagious, caused by a particular pathogen. The process here is that a pathogen finds a particularly inviting host, settles in and stays dormant. The body is either unable to detect it and ward it off at the entry point, but detects it, once it has settled in the tissues. Then, it attacks it, but its weapons are so crude that it ends up attacking its own tissues. It also happens because pathogens are very good at drilling deep inside the cells, interweaving their bodies and genetic material with ours, and often masking themselves as our own.

Another manifestation of immune response to pathogens, as well as other problems like vitamin deficiencies, presence of toxins, irritants, any kind of damage or intrusion, is depositing materials to patch up the problem, or insulate the body from the element. Calcium is a common material that body uses to isolate itself from perceived physical intruders, or—pathogens. One can find its deposits all over the body. A strange and rare phenomenon that has happened in history—was when a woman in Morocco was pregnant but never gave birth to her child. The child was found inside her, completely calcified, in a form of a huge egg, about 50 years later.

Cholesterol build up appears to be patching up tiny tears that are similar to those that people get on the skin, suggesting that eczema and psoriasis can occur anywhere in the body, including the inner walls of blood vessels. It is analogous to keloid scars that take over the site of the original tissue damage, in an inflamed reaction. In my visual modeling, Alzheimer's falls in the same category, where the myelin sheath of neurons is damaged with scars, when the body goes overboard in attacking a pathogen, living in those neurons.

In sum, through my modeling, I see most auto-immune diseases as caused by either viruses or some other smaller and harder to detect particles. Maybe they are virulent proteins? But it is something very similar to our own cells, or it knows how to hide very well, and that is why the body has a hard time differentiating them from its own material.

So, who really done it?

I propose that virtually all diseases of modern times, which we call incurable, or idiopathic, are caused by pathogens, either known or still unknown to us. There is nothing bad about a pathogen. A pathogen is only seen as a pathogen and a hostile agent because it causes an undesirable symptom. Only then do we try to either kill it off or make it permanently inactive, and that in itself we define as a true cure, as opposed to temporarily suppressing the negative effects of its activity.

Causes can be inferred from the treatments that work to assuage a disease. If we look at causes of a disease as a combination of factors, then a successful remedy must be affecting one of those factors. If we look at the holistic medicine remedies for most incurable diseases, such as diabetes,

Alzheimer's, asthma, COPD, arthritis and cancer, we will see that they all contain anti-bacterial and anti-viral remedies. Curiously, a list of remedies for inflammation always appear to contain an antibacterial/antiviral agent. Some remedies only suppress the symptoms—they are diuretics, antihistamines, steroids... But an antibacterial/antiviral agent is just that—it kills or deactivates bacteria and viruses. If it succeeds in stopping or suppressing the disease, it means that bacteria and viruses are present, and de facto are causing the disease.

Think of chemotherapy for cancer, for example. Why is it that these remedies for incurable diseases are all geared toward killing a pathogen? It may be because these diseases are all caused by pathogens that we have not yet discovered, so we are still failing to pinpoint what they are. Once we discover these pathogens, we can target them more precisely and not destroy so much of our native tissues, along with them, as it happens in chemotherapy.

If we see the cause of diseases as a combination of pathogens and a weak immune system, then we can either target the pathogens, or try to make the immune system stronger, or both. If the causing pathogen is unknown or poorly understood, we can try to strengthen the immune system—which is the case with COVID-19, a virus that has devastated the world in the year 2020. However, isolating the pathogens, in addition to making the immune system stronger, is very is a hundredfold more powerful, as it will alleviate the need to fight them, lowering the stress load on our immune system.

Medical researchers have to search and find these disease-causing pathogens, isolate them, and construct a lethal weapon, specific for each one, so as to come up with a cure. But before that happens, we can also do something to protect ourselves, primarily by strengthening our immune system.

Viruses and fungi as farmers of bacteria.

The most terrifying vision that has surfaced over and over again, as I have modeled the activity of pathogens, is that they appear to be aware of each other! Some of them fight each other, some have an ongoing vendetta, some use others as a guide to where the grass is greener, and many have developed symbiotic relationships of abuse and exploitation. It is quite bizarre, but what I have seen is that viruses often manipulate bacteria, as if bacteria were their farm animals! I have also seen pernicious fungi sending out scouts to look for good places to establish new settlements in human bodies!

Viruses appear to have a vicious and unscrupulous collective mind, regarding everything as a fair game—even the fungi. In fact, viruses appear to be farming bacteria for all kinds of purposes! One is to maintain good feeding grounds for themselves.

Sugar to bacteria is what gold is to humans. Bacteria are always on the lookout for sugar, and this has everything to do with obesity, with diabetes, with cellulite, and with estrogen, it turns out! Bacteria attack inflamed and toxic tissues, and viruses follow them, infect the host and make the environment even friendlier to the bacteria, so that the bacteria would multiply, feast on the body, and keep it weak, without killing it. Killing the body would mean the end of a settlement for both viruses and bacteria, so only those who keep the body sustainably sick and alive, are the ones who have survived in the competition. Isn't it funny that in most diseases we know, viral infections are usually accompanied by bacterial infections—even during flu!

There are many methods viruses use to keep the sugar in the body for the bacteria. Sugar can be consumed directly from many of its forms, primarily glucose, but also derived from fat. One thing that viruses do is increase the size of fat cells—as in cellulite and obesity. That way, the human host can retain more fat, since the number of fat cells stops increasing at adulthood. Then, bacteria settle in the fat and feast on it. Another thing they do is invade the pancreas and disrupt the insulin function—as in diabetes, both type A and B. Since insulin would make sure that the extra sugar is ousted from the body, viruses do everything to deactivate this hormone. There is one absolutely abhorrent practice that I have observed: viruses act as drug dealers with bacteria: they hook bacteria onto sugar, and then have them begging for a dose, and in return— bacteria do what they are told. In human terms, it is human trafficking, but chemically that is exactly what it looks like! Finally, viruses also cause increased estrogen production, because estrogen increases fat retention in the body. Those are just a few of the cunning ways that viruses make sure that bacteria have sugar to feast on, so that the viruses have a comfortable place for active existence.

Viruses are not the only pathogens who farm bacteria: mushroom also use them in similar ways. Mushrooms are extremely intelligent, and have a hierarchical internal group organization. They appear to be using both bacteria and viruses for their predatory scavenging. The first disease that has shown me this picture was cancer. Cancer appears to be caused by a fungus that works with both bacteria and viruses. The host must be weak and act as a friendly environment for bacteria, then viruses follow, and only then the fungi take over to finish up and devoir the host. If it were only bacteria and viruses, people would not be dying from cancer at the same rate as they are.

Diseases that have lethal outcomes seem to be curated by fungi, and the chronic ones that make humans suffer but not die—do not seem to involve all three working together. Of course, people die from bacterial and viral infections, but statistically—that is a minuscule number compared to the cases when all three pathogens are working symbiotically. If one could zoom into the microcosm of the micro-world, one would be stupefied at the number and variety of pathogens devouring the host, at the peak of a disease. Humans appear to be living cadavers, barely seen behind the pathogens that devoir them alive.

Sugar, salt, and iodine.

Sugar would not be so bad for us, if it were not gold in the world of bacteria. The only reason sugar is poison to us is because it is food for our main enemy —the pathogens. Sugar would not make us gain weight anywhere near as much, if it were not for the pathogens who used us as a sugar plantation!

Salt is not bad for us, as some people claim in sweeping generalizations. Salt both increases edema, which makes the toxins less poisonous in the mixture, and creates an unfriendly environment for the bacteria. There is a reason that Dead Sea is called dead—because its high concentration of salt ensures that its water contains virtually no bacteria. Some people crave salt, especially those with diseased liver, and sometimes that may be for a good reason: their body is telling them that there is an overgrowth of bacteria that must be combatted.

Even the thyroid function is involved with bacteria eating us! Curiously iodine is a common antibacterial, and the lack of it generally causes hypothyroidism—a lowered thyroid function. This antibacterial pattern of behavior is present is an overwhelming number of bodily functions, as they relate to diseases. Substances that affect bacteria also interfere with viruses and fungi in our body, because those usually work together in some way.

Waves and pathogens.

There is something interesting to be said about how all pathogens are affected by sound, radio, and other types of waves,—and they are greatly affected! That may be a major factor in why some people are less susceptible to diseases than others. Waves change the chemical environment by making it more or less friendly for pathogens, and can be either produced internally by the brain or come from the external world. Brain waves are still poorly understood, and in my modeling, they keep coming up as essential in controlling diseases. The emotional experience of will power and determination seems to cause the brain to produce brainwaves that prevent pathogens from settling in. Feelings of hatred, envy, and guild—do the opposite: they signal for pathogens to come in. I can clearly see it in my visualizations.

As for the external waves, there are so many different ones that it is hard to say which ones function in which way. However, harmony seems to have a positive effect, and cacophony—negative. The majority of artificially created objects emit inaudible cacophony, harmful to humans. I can actually hear a lot of the waves that should not be heard—those produced by electrical devices, for example. And this electric noise that surrounds us—chronically abuses our immune system, affecting our tissues and liquids on the atomic and cellular level, and attracts pathogens to our bodies, by creating imperceptible inflammation in the tissues. Pathogens are also attracted to certain waves, and also structures that those waves create in liquids. There is really a lot of value in studies on structured water, and how it affects human health.

Contagious antibodies?

There is another fascinating realization has emerged from modeling how pathogens attacks humans: not only are pathogens contagious, but also that something that knows how to fight them back. It appears that there is a contagious substance that carries information on how to fight pathogens. If a group of people all get sick with the same disease, and one of the members develops a mechanism to fight them back, the rest of the group are likely to catch it. Thus, as the disease spreads, the anti-disease also spreads, and the chances of someone having developed just the right contagious anti-bodies, that can be communally shared, also increases. It looks like living in groups of close proximity, such as families, has an evolutionary advantage in that, besides transferring contagious diseases, it also allows to transfer the knowledge of how to fight them back, so the group can survive. Yes, I know that it sounds zany, but that is what my visual modeling keeps showing!

Vitamins and nutrition.

Vitamin deficiency is something we can easily control by eating foods with high vitamin content, and supplementing our diet with food-sourced vitamins. Because of totality of chemical processes is too complex to fathom in its entirety by a human being, supplementing with multi-vitamins, plus those specific to each person's needs,—is the best policy, and it takes effort to discover the individually optimal list and dosage. The scope of this topic is well beyond the scope of this little book, but it is a good start to realize that we are all malnourished and starving for vitamins. Eating something just to quench our hunger is deadly, eating something solely for pleasure—as well. We first must limit what we eat to foods high in nutrition, and then choose combinations we find good to taste. Otherwise, we waste our energy digesting substances that do not benefit us nutritionally, and do nothing to build our immune system. It is like putting in water instead of gas into your car and hope that it runs.

The role of toxins.

Toxins weaken us, making us send out SOS signals, to which pathogens are highly attuned. From the point of view of pathogens, I t reminds me of Californian Gold Rush of the nineteenth century, when someone discovered gold, and the rumors of it attracted tens of thousands of workers, all trying to get rich.

Just like rumors of gold spread all over the world, presence of toxins, and the chemical damage they do to human tissues, serve as a direct message to pathogens, who have learned that presence of a certain toxin carries a high likelihood of there being inflammation and weakened cells to attack. Avoiding toxins in the first place is the best preventative measure, but detoxing one's body is a also an indispensable, yet traumatic, process, both of which are crucial in the battle against pathogens.

Stress causes toxins to be produced by the body, and one can either cut that process in the bud by eliminating sources of stress, or catch it later, after the toxins are already there—by leading them out of the body.

Certainly, books and books have been written about how to detoxify, how to destress, what diet to choose, and what vitamins to take. People are used to treating disease with a particular medicine to either suppress a symptom, or to kill a pathogen. Yet, even if we discover all of the unknown pathogens and find specific cures for each one of them, the need for a strong immune system will never be obviated, because it protects us from everything, known and unknown.

Zany cures for the incurable.

Etiology is the study of the causes of a disease. If we entertain the idea that most currently incurable diseases are caused by pathogens, we can make a thought experiment, and see what natural remedies already exist for them. If those remedies have something to do with destroying bacteria, viruses, and fungi—there is a clue in support of the pathogen hypothesis.

These are some of the incurable diseases that affect modern humanity:

Allergies, alopecia, asthma, vitiligo, fibromyalgia, arthritis, autism, eczema and psoriasis, Irritable Bowel Syndrome, myopia, COPD, Carpal Tunnel, diabetes, polycystic syndrome in ovaries, cancer, migraine, schizophrenia.

Cure is something that eliminates the disease and does not require any more subsequent actions. There are various medicines that curb the symptoms or stifle the development of these diseases, but there is still no true cure for any of them. Looking at all these diseases through the hypothesis of pathogenic invasion gives hope to finding a cure for all of them. All it takes is finding the pathogen that causes the disease and finding a chemical weapon to kill it off. It is difficult, but it is a great deal easier than not knowing at all what enemy to fight, and in which direction. There could be a cluster of pathogens working together, any possible combination of viruses, bacteria, fungi, etc.

Many of the incurable diseases manifest themselves in an allergic reaction of the body to the pathogen. So, it is not pathogen itself who does the damage, but the reaction of the human body, as it is trying to eliminate the pathogen. All types of allergies are precisely that, according to my modeling. One possible cause of an immune reaction is simply an unknown pathogen. An interesting element in the equation is that some substances only appear similar to the pathogens the body has been previously exposed to. So, when that substance is consumed, the body reacts to it as if it were a pathogen it already knows, and increases its reaction with repeated offense. Yet another possibility is that a certain food, contaminated with a pathogen, was consumed and caused inflammation once. Then, the food became associated with the pathogen, and under repeated exposure, the body started reacting to it with an attack. In the case of peanut butter allergy, it could be that peanut butter is contaminated with a pathogen current medical science does not recognize, or it could be that something in it mimics a pathogen that some bodies have been exposed to, or a person has previously consumed contaminated peanut butter, and their body has forever remembered this traumatic experience.

Kinds of dirt.

In addition, it seems that people living in a dirty urban environment have more allergies than people living in rural environments with minimal amenities, in what would be considered dirty by the developed world. The matter is that there are different kinds of dirt. Natural dirt that comes from animal and human bodies simply living—in nature, is washed out by the elements like rain, wind, and the sun. The types of pathogens that are found there have evolved over millennia to not harm humans— with the new exceptions of animal viruses crossing into the human world. Urban environments are not filtered, cleared and washed the same way as rural ones, because they lack natural drainage systems. They are not washed and disinfected by the rain, wind and the sun, but rely on people doing the cleaning. People are very bad at cleaning, compared to nature. Sprung upon toxic artificial materials, pathogens that grow in dirty urban environments are relatively new to humans, they have been produced in the closed system conditions, and humans have not yet developed immunity to them. It appears to me that spending time in a rural environment is beneficial for people from the city, because it is there that the immune system will learn different types of defenses that might make it stronger even in the face of pathogens that grow in the cities.

Going further with the theme of allergic reactions, it appears in my modeling that autoimmune diseases are essentially allergies, and, just like allergies, are caused by a yet unknown pathogen.

Some notes on the diseases.

All of the incurable diseases mentioned below seem to be caused by a pathogen, and if one looks at the holistic remedies that help against them—one will see that they all have an antibacterial or antiviral component.

Arthritis.

Arthritis is usually treated with medications that suppress the immune function, and thus prevent the body from attacking itself, causing pain and discomfort of the joints. This only partially eliminates the unpleasant symptoms, at the expense of opening up one's body to all existing diseases and pathogens. Holistic medicine suggests herbal remedies such as boswellia, turmeric, cat's claw, and others,—all of which are antibacterial, anti-viral, or anti-fungal. What's amazing is that they work! What's even more amazing is that the same herbal remedies work for all of these incurable diseases. Notice a pattern? If they all tend to work on all of the incurable diseases, and they all are targeting pathogens, there   must be something to it.

Alzheimer's.

Alzheimer's is an inflammation of the brain tissues, and inflammation itself is a sign of an infection—at least, in my world of disease modeling. That is, when physical and direct chemical abuse is excluded. Nothing has access to the brain, except what can pass through the blood-brain barrier, and that could very well be pathogens. Yerba Santa, an antibacterial, is said to help with Alzheimer's, and what is it also used for traditionally? On asthma! And also on tuberculosis, common colds, and bronchitis, all of which are known to be caused by pathogenic bacteria. It could also be that the culprit is a virus, but by killing the bacteria that this virus is farming, we cut off its life supply.

Vitiligo.

When the human body attacks the melanin-producing cells that give skin color, people get those bright white patches on their skin. Everyone says they are not contagious. Maybe they are not contagious via skin-to-skin contact, or under other circumstances, but the cause of this disease appears to me to be pathogens, which are contagious by their very nature. There must be a place the people contracted that pathogen that selected pigment-producing cells as their host, and now the body is attacking those cells with doses of homemade chemotherapy, killing them wholesale, because it is unable to isolate and target the pathogen directly. One of vitiligo treatments is bearberry, which is an antibacterial—once again.

Eczema and psoriasis.

The story here is the same as with vitiligo, except different kind of cells are chosen as a host for the pathogen, and so the symptoms differ slightly, when the body attacks those cells. Treatments for both eczema and psoriasis consist of antibacterial and anti-viral agents, in combination with those for body detoxification. Once again, it follows the pattern of treating a pathogen or a cluster of pathogens, in complex with eliminating toxins that create a friendly environment for them.

Autism.

One small observation that I was able to make during my years of teaching at the American high schools, where I was able to observe thousands of children with autism: their parents tend to have auto-immune disorders, such as eczema and psoriasis, which are visible to the naked eye and do not require any special investigation. I noticed it with such great frequency among this particular group that I could not dismiss it as purely coincidental. My brain instantly modeled the diseases, and gave out an answer to me that autism is caused by a pathogen that settles in some brain tissue, and then the child's body attacks it. Apparently, this pathogen is able to cross the blood-brain barrier.

Interestingly enough, the controversies regarding vaccines causing autism do appear to have some merit. According to my modeling, autistic children were infected by autism-causing pathogens through contaminated vaccines, or through their parents, who were contaminated first. Some children's or parents' immune systems did not develop a severe auto-immune reaction to those pathogens, and some did. Those who did— developed autism. It looks like the rate of contamination is low, and the rate of immune reactions is also relatively low. Otherwise, many more children have been exposed to these autism-causing pathogens then the number of those who actually developed the symptoms.

Diabetes.

Diabetes deserves a special mention, because it is so closely connected to the gold that bacteria are after—sugar. The reason drastic weight loss and liposuction tend to improve diabetes condition is because they remove huge parts of fat—the home of the bacterial colonies that are farming sugar in us, and are in turn, being farmed by viruses and maybe even fungus. Both types of diabetes tend to run in families, and natural sugar-stabilizing remedies are largely anti-bacterial, like turmeric, gotu kola, and berberine.

Irritable Bowel Syndrome.

We are poorly protected against pathogens, physically speaking. They can enter our body through our mouth, nose, eyes, ears, genitals, and even through skin. Mouth, however, is the main pathway, simply because of the frequency of direct exposure to pathogens of all kinds when we eat. We literally ingest pounds of parasites, bacteria, viruses, and non-food particles, just in one single year of our life.

If the mouth does not have enough enzymes to break down some pathogens and enough saliva to flush them down, they can proliferate right there, settling on any tissue, and in the crevices between teeth, causing caries. Stomach has bile, which is acid that kills most pathogens, if there is enough of it produced. Quite commonly, there is not enough bile to kill all of the pathogens, or it is just not chemically equipped to do so, and so they spread along our gut, all the way to the anus. They also seep into the rest of our body. Candida is one awful example!

That greatly diminishes our ability to digest food and absorb the nutrients, while pathogens irritate the lining, producing inflammation. Further, our immune system attacks our stomach and gut, creating even more inflammation, and there arise the symptoms, which all together, are called Irritable Bowel Syndrome, and a slew of other related diseases. Predictably now, such diseases are treated with anti-bacterial, anti-viral, anti-fungal, and anti-parasitic agents, because any combination of them could be the culprit.

Schizophrenia, epilepsy, and migraines.

A common symptom that accompanies migraines is brain tissue swelling and inflammation—the two most common symptoms of infection, and what bacteria, viruses, and fungi are attracted to. In my visualizations, many of the diseases of the brain turn out to be caused by pathogens, even though a complex of symptoms that surround them can point to all kinds of other causes, including precipitation of waste materials that have not been washed away due to lack of sleep, for example. That is just toxins that signal pathogens to come over, and create a friendly environment for them to settle. One widely discussed natural remedy against schizophrenia is ashwagandha—an herb with strong anti-bacterial properties. It is that same pathogen trail, again.

Cancer.

Cancer spreads exactly like the humans have been spreading all over the planet—like a giant fungal network of settlements. Humanity to the planet Earth is essentially what cancer is to a human body. Cancer sends out its scouts all around, looking for sugar, acidity, and inflammation, which are all signs of disease and weakness,—an easy feast for the cancerous mushroom to settle in. Sugar—because bacteria eat it, after a virus has manipulated insulin and caused the cells to not absorb it, so it stays "on the loose" and available. Acidity—because where there are bacteria, there is their waste, which is acidic, which signals to the cancer that there are decaying or inflamed tissues to feast on. Inflammation is a perfect ground for feasting.

How is inflammation signaled? Sometimes acidity, and sometimes—there are other chemical signs which I don't know yet. How is cancer spread? Through air, through skin contact, through liquids. It is the most spreadable and the most contagious of all diseases. However, when more of it is present at a certain place, it becomes more contagious, due to its possible quorum sensing—when its collective mind feels more numerous, more powerful, more capable, and, therefore, more decisive in its attacks. One thing is clear to me: cancer spores are everywhere! Some places have more of them, some—less.

We probably have all survived more than a single cancer attack during our lifetimes, without even knowing it. Cancer is a definite scavenger, and any sickness or weakness in the body, including toxins, emotional stress, and physical injury is a fair game. Because of it, there are a myriad of factors that influence whether one is overtaken by cancer: good bacteria in the gut, positive emotions, detoxification, unfriendly environment for pathogens (salt, sun UV rays, apple cider vinegar, structured water, avoidance of known allergens), and many-many more.

One curious factor with cancer is human susceptibility to it, when under emotional stress, or even sadness. Chronic feelings of guilt, envy, jealousy, hatred, of being unloved, disrespected, unappreciated, gaslit, and exposure to narcissists—all set a human being at high risk of cancer. I see humans turn dark in color under emotional duress, and they even smell different: somehow rotten, nauseatingly sweet, and or rancid. Surely, they smell attractive and inviting to all kinds of cancers on the prowl.

How to get protected.

The good news for us is that, because a disease is a complex meeting of several factors, it is enough that we upset one single factor, in order to either prevent a disease from happening, or to stop it, once it has started. We turn to the health formula, where we find these four major factors: pathogens, vitamins, toxins, and stress.

Protecting ourselves against disease-causing pathogens has all to do with making ourselves less attractive as a host. After all, even sharks attack the weakest seal, just like tigers attack the weakest gazelle. So do pathogens with humans: they are the predators, stocking our human flock, preying on the weakest: those with compromised immune system, the young, and the old. Yet, it is not the age that makes us attractive to them, but particular chemical messages that our bodies send to communicate with the pathogenic world outside.

Independent of pathogens, we can do a lot with ourselves, to make us less attractive to them. It is the same as acting a certain way, so as to ward of serial killers, on the lookout for potential prey. It is also the same as being stuck in a jungle, full of flesh-eating predators, and disguising yourself as a green leaf. This is what many animals do in nature, in order to survive, and so can we.

Vitamins, avoidance of pathogens, toxins and stress are crucial in disease prevention. Each of the four factors has its particular loopholes. With the exception of pathogens, they all have to do with strengthening one's immune system. There are many types of pathogens: bacteria, viruses, fungi, mycoplasma bacteria that can behave like mushrooms, misfolded proteins, just plain parasites, and many others that remain yet undiscovered. All of them are after us: we provide them with bed and breakfast, which are free and mostly sustainable. What we can do is avoid being exposed to them in high concentrations. Being exposed to pathogens makes our body react by going into a stressful state, changing us chemically, which makes our bodies tired and weakened, and consequently, starts us sending out chemical messages of being a better target for pathogens.

However, there is no need to panic and avoid going into the public and being afraid that a slightest contact with a pathogen will cause disease. Surely, being exposed to a lot of pathogens at a time can cause their quorum sensing mechanism to entertain an idea that you are a good host: merely by there being enough of them relative to the strength of your immune system. Yet, not any public space is automatically dangerous. Places with higher concentrations are closed spaces with a lot of people, especially if the ventilation is poor. So, working in a hospital, where one is exposed to high concentrations of pathogens, especially over a period of time, is one of the ways to increase risk of this happening. Gyms and public transportation are less risky. The highest risk of exposure is one's home, if there is a sick person living there.

I don't know exactly the chemical that makes pathogens sense human chemical distress remotely, but inflammation, edema, and a whole slew of condition and symptoms give off chemical messages, far and wide, signaling to the pathogens whether they are a good prospect. Pathogens literally smell us and our chemical makeup, and will always go for an easy kill.

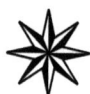

LONGEVITY

There is no cure for death, but one can postpone it, which in itself is a cure, if only a temporary one. Each human has a story arc: birth, youth, middle age, and the wane phase. Yet, the nature doesn't, it is forever young. Every morning, the sun comes up, all pure and innocent, as if whatever happened yesterday meant nothing. It constantly washes and renews itself, and if we can copycat it, at least, in some things, maybe we can keep winning over death for much longer than we have in the past.

Blaming disease on old age is like saying that somebody died because they were born. Diseases do not come with mere age, they all have specific causes, external to our body,—except maybe telomeres that protect our DNA from deterioration and control our cellular renewal.

Factors prolonging life.

Briefly, if you don't do anything else, the main three rules for longevity are resting only when you are tired, eating only when you hungry, and drinking only when you are thirsty. It applies to every activity, and the gist of it is doing everything in its right time. The challenge for everyone is to figure out when that right time is. However, there is much more.

What I am about to tell you can't hurt, but it may help. It certainly has helped me, but there is still time to test its centennial efficiency. It is a compilation of notes from my observations of people living long lives, all over the world, filtered through my ideasthetic visualization. This is what they seem to have in common, besides what we all already know.

Cleanliness.

People who live long lives tend to have better personal hygiene, or they simply live in natural environments, where nature cleans them and itself.

Some people have a terrible habit of putting things in their mouth, just to hold them. That is a perfect invitation for all kinds of pathogens to enter the body. Washing one's hands immediately upon entering home from outside is a great habit to have!

Brushing one's teeth twice a day is a dire necessity, so as to get rid of pathogens that, by the way, are eating you raw, if you don't get them out of there. They are not only eating your soft tissues, but they are burrowing into the enamel of your teeth—that is how people get cavities. Scraping off the tongue is important too, because, if you zoom in, you will see a jungle of trees with thick branches. They look more like seaweed, really, but the flora and fauna there—will blow your mind! Some of it is good for you, but a lot of it is enemies that need to be eliminated. Rinsing with a solution of hydrogen peroxide or some other antibacterial and anti-fungal liquid is the best defense. Xylitol gum works great, too.

Pathogens hiding in people's homes is a big topic. Here are some basics. The counters, sinks, floors, and other surfaces should be regularly cleaned, because you are acting out the role of rain, sun, and wind at home—those that would do all the cleaning in nature. I wipe counters, door and faucet handles, and even keys with rubbing alcohol. Sinks and tubs get disinfected with bleach, and floors can be washed either with bleach or some other soapy agent. Sheets should be washed at least once in two weeks, in hot water, and blankets and pillows—dried in the drier every few months. The home has to be aired out as much as possible. Optimally, the windows would not ever close. And even "more optimally", we would all be living under the open sky, which would eliminate all these artificially created problems! These are best practices, but anything approximating this cleaning regime will do wonders to your health.

Exercise.

People who live long lives generally don't overexert themselves. There are many others who go into extremes, when trying to improve themselves, and it certainly applies to exercising. According to my modeling, exercising when one is tired is detrimental to health. Exercise seems to be best when one is full of pent up energy, burning to come out. Not letting it out is bad for health, and letting it out is the exercise that is most beneficial to both and mind.

During exercise, it is best to be right at the top of the distribution curve: don't work too hard, and don't slack off either. Slacking off will not refresh your body to the full potential, and working too hard will actually damage it. Exercising on the fresh air is best, just because it is cleaner than indoors, if it is in the nature, and because of all the "nutrients" that fresh air contains, especially when one is surrounded by lush greenery.

Some of the best exercises are fast walking, dancing, and swimming, because they are not repetitive, they work on most of the human muscles, and have a strong element of enjoyment—which is crucial for longevity. Walking on flat surfaces is harmful to the bones, because it puts repetitive pressure on the same small points in the body. Walking on surfaces that are uneven, like paths in the forest or on sand, distributes pressure and tension throughout the whole body, exercising many muscles at varied intervals, and gently energizing the entire person.

It is really a tug of war. In each human, there are two opposing forces, pulling in opposite directions: one is pacifying, and the other—exhilarating. When you feel like being active and jumping around—just do it. When you feel like resting—lay down and take a nap. It is important to please each force, at the right time. If you let one of them win over the other—you get old, or even become sick. When the pacifying force is winning, the person stagnates. When the exhilarating force is winning—person is warn out and exhausted. Neither one is good or bad in itself: it is all about keeping a balance, an equilibrium between the two. When you are tired—rest, when you are full of energy—spend it.

Finally, sweating is good for longevity, and one should not be afraid of it if one wants to live a long life.

Emotional balance.

If you have not yet noticed, many people who live to a hundred, live in rural, underdeveloped areas, with barely any amenities. That also means a lack of modern stressors like technology, traffic, noise, notifications and constant news. That also means a very steady emotional state, with few ups and downs to wear the person down.

On the other hand, in our modern world, it is fashionable to be excited about everything, whether good or bad. As a society, we have decided that everything must be intense, and it has made us pay the price with years, deducted from our lives. We work hard and party hard, we multi-task and speed through everything. If someone is not worried, they are considered irresponsible. If someone is not busy, they negatively regarded as unproductive. I know that in the complex world in which we live, those things are a must, but I do hope that someday we can figure out how to change our prescribed lifestyle, so that we could live longer.

In addition, if things get too calm and relaxing, we seek out excitement. We are addicted to negative news, we love to hate, and we actually subconsciously crave for something to upset us, so that we can put up a fight and see what happens. These days, people expose themselves to all kinds of danger, just to feel alive: from bungee jumping, to free-falling from an airplane, to watching horror films. Another sad proof of our love for sensations is clear when people take out their cell phones to record an act of violence, instead of coming to help. They know that their recording will produce the same excitement they are feeling right now, again and again, and their anticipation of pleasure overpowers any moral calling.

Bad news, although negative, are actually addictive because they all cause an emotional spike that in small doses feels like pleasure, if one is otherwise bored. In addition, when the brain detected potential danger and harm, it pumps you with painkillers big time! Liking bad news is exactly like being addicted to painkillers, addicted to prescribed drugs! We are not addicted to the bad news, but to the happy chemicals our brains produce, in order to help us weather those bad news.

All this extraordinary excitement costs us years of life. Some people will gladly pay this price, so this is just for your information.

Comfort food.

Comfort food is a concept that applies to far more things than just food. It is the Danish word hygge—all about feeling safe, loved, and comfortable. With our Neo-nomadic lifestyle, we have very little of it, and whole industries feed off our longing for it. We are not only vitamin-deficient, but we are critically oxytocin deficient. There is even a saying that actors die from being under-praised, and regular people die from being under-loved. Those who live long lives, usually live in small and stable communities, where they receive large amounts of oxytocin by being sure of reciprocal love and support, and where they are surrounded by trust, safety, and certainty.

In fact, avoiding toxic people, who destroy our emotional safety and balance, and even those who stand you up on appointments, and those upon whom you cannot rely to keep their word, will lengthen your life.

Sleep.

People who live long lives tend to go to sleep early and wake up early, and take an afternoon nap. No frills, simple as that. When they get tired, they don't drink coffee to dehydrate and coerce their body to action, when it is screaming to let it rest. Yes, they sleep whenever they get tired—a virtually impossible luxury for anyone in the developed world.

Sleeping in complete darkness is less common in developed societies, where lights are everywhere, even by diffusion. Yet, it is crucial in regulation of the circadian rhythms and production of melatonin, which literally controls our wellbeing.

Sleeping on harder surfaces promotes longevity, and it might be because it allows the muscles to relax during sleep, because they don't have to stay tense to keep the body in one integrated piece—the hard surface does it for them. That way, the distant between vertebrae can stay wider, and those spaces will stay replenished with fluid, preventing the commonly recognized shrinkage that happens with age, and allowing free flow of nutrients.

In fact, in my modeling, the reason our joints crack has nothing to do with the official version, which states that gas bubbles between bones are released upon chiropractic manipulations and it is they who cause the cracking sound. My modeling has shown me, thousands of times, that the sound of cracking comes from tiny suction cups being popped of. It also shows me that, in addition to the muscles holding our body together, the bones have tiny suction cups that temporarily attach them to each other, so as to help the muscles, especially, when one has to carry a heavy weight. So, when our bones crack, we actually hear millions of tiny suction cups popping, as they are being unstuck from surfaces. Maybe we inherited it from Neanderthals? Just kidding. Or not. Well, I don't know. But Neanderthals are known to be extremely robust and well built to carry heavy weights, so I got that little inkling in my mind.

Pleasure.

People who live longer lives experience less guilt and more pleasure in their lives. That is by no means meant to encourage psychopathic behavior. Those people actually live in conditions with widely available healthy sources of pleasure, like enjoying the simple things in life, like enjoying being vulnerable to friends and relatives, and almost absent competition among peers. Not all sources of pleasure are equally beneficial. Altruistic behavior, respecting one's self because of good deeds, wishing others well, enjoying arts and music, seeking out beauty in life in general—are the most powerful life-prolonging pleasures. Such pleasures greatly lengthen life, but displeasure, such as disappointment in one's moral stature, disgust, envy, hatred, and guilt—drastically cut it down.

It seems that feeling guilty is much less common in simple societies, because their life is not so fraught with temptations and social competition, and there are not as many reasons to do things for which one will end up feeling embarrassed. The challenge for those living in complex and dynamic societies is to find a social nest where one feels optimally safe and certain of their surroundings, and is exposed to minimal predicaments. Finally, enjoying simple things is possible anywhere on earth.

Laziness.

People who live longer lives do not tend to be lazy. On the contrary, they tend to have a great willpower, self-discipline, and inner strength, where the word "must" carries a much greater weight that the word "want." They tend to be hard workers: mentally and physically.

In all of my modeling, I have never seen laziness to come out as a cause of strengthening of human body, except when people go into extremes and overexert themselves, when they should be resting. It might be something psychosomatic, but willpower works wonders.

Singing.

People who sing tend to live longer. It may have to do with many factors, but what stands out for me is sustained prolonged breathing that is required for singing and the sound waves that somehow affect the water content in our bodies. In addition, singing often takes place in groups, as in choirs, and the comradery in the musical environment is extremely nurturing.

Celebration.

People who celebrate regularly appear to live longer. And it is celebrating in a traditional way, with all the solemn awareness of the event and its passage, with all the faith in its importance. Interestingly, people who believe in ancient rituals, such as coming of age, marriage, and burial rites, actually appear less worried and sure of themselves and their future. It may be that rituals do have an important function in our wellbeing: they provide a framework of certainty and trust in others and what tomorrow might bring.

Diet.

It turns out that people with the greatest protein intake live the longest, everything else being equal. It may be that eating more protein forces people to eat fewer carbohydrates, and promotes production of ketones that are superior for sustainable energy than sugar. Actually, that is what makes people different from bacteria who function on sugar! And, don't ask me why, but here I once again see a link to Neanderthals: the more Neanderthal DNA one has, the more urgent is their need of protein for longevity. Zany, isn't it? I am only reporting what I see.

It turns out that social eating does not promote good health, but only if it means active talking and being overly emotionally involved in the conversation. Two things are disrupted by overspecializing during meals: chewing for long enough to macerate and predigest the food, and stomach relaxation, so that it is ready accept the food for digestion. We actually fall into a fight-or-flight mode during intense socializing, which goes as far as blocking bile from flowing in order to digest food.

It turns out that smoothies are only good for us, if we actively chew them, before sending them down to the stomach. Otherwise, they don't go through the essential pre-digestion stage, and so are less likely to be well digested in the stomach, and their nutrients absorbed. And, there is more: eating with one's hands is also good for longevity: it is not only comforting, but it also sends signals to the stomach about the texture and temperature of the food one is about to eat. What else?

Freshness in food is crucial, which means absolutely no leftovers! You catch it or pick it, then you cook it, you eat it, and that's the end of it. Otherwise, bacteria start growing in that food, as it decomposes, even if slowly and invisibly to a human eye. That, in turn brings in pathogens and toxins straight into our body.

Finally, Asia seems to have gotten it right: hot, liquid food is much better for longevity than dry and cold. Plus, all tastes, including sour and bitter, are good for humans. It is not all about sweets. And spices, largely neglected in the West, are surprisingly powerful in prolonging one's life.

Finally, all these diets and prolonged fasting, as well as excluding one type of food or another— they don't appear to correlate with longevity. Moderation is the magic word here, and it is all about finding the golden middle. There are rules of thumb to follow: eating only when one is hungry, eating hot and liquid, and eating a little of everything, without going into extremes in any direction. That means eating everything, and excluding nothing from one's diet. That means eating 2-3 times a day, starting with a big breakfast. Fasting for prolonged periods of time interferes with bile production and causes bacterial overgrowth in the gut, eating too often interferes with insulin function and prevents proper digestion.

Sun exposure.

Finally, people who live longer spend more time outdoors and out on the sun. My modeling shows that skin cancer is not caused by the sun, but by pathogens who reside in the skin. When the sun even slightly damages the skin tissues, those pathogens activate and attack. Strangely enough, the sun actually kills pathogens, too.

It may be that, with people spending a lot of time outdoors, continuous sun exposure never allows pathogens to grow in number in the first place, to the point where they could feel confident to attack. People who spend most time indoors often lack Vitamin D, which regulates the entire immune system, and so pathogens are much more likely to prosper in their bodies. Once those people come out onto the sun, the pathogens are already great in number, the skin is not used to sun exposure, gets irritated, and the pathogens attack, causing cancer.

Salt, high altitude, and water.

People who live near the sea tend to live longer. People who live high in the mountains also live longer than average. But those who regularly swim in salty water, in the seas and oceans, also live longer than the rest. It is hard to compare proximity to water, to high altitude, to salt baths, as factors in longevity, but they all appear to prolong life. Living near the sea could be calming, or it could infuse the air people breath with negative ions, or the air might be naturally anti-bacterial, containing salt particles. High altitude might exert the body just the right way, making it work harder to pump oxygen to the tissues, and also might benefit humans with exceptional purity of air.

Benefits of swimming in salt are more immediately noticeable: salty water acts as a diuretic, counteracting edema, which is already a good sign. Salt is anti-bacterial: this is what they use to preserve meats, after all. As we swim, salty water penetrates our skin and seeps into our body, which is bound to suppress pathogen growth.

On a good note.

Yes, we are slowly decomposing every day. However, the good news is, we are much more in control of our decomposition than we think. Remember, will power is one of the greatest powers a human has, and it is this will that will cure our way to longevity.

BEAUTY

They say, old age is incurable. But you can still live to be a hundred, and then die beautiful. And suddenly, the adage "Live long, die young!" no longer sounds like an oxymoron!

Everything that makes someone healthy, also makes them beautiful. In fact, in my ideasthetic mental modeling and research, it looks like health is the main determinant in being perceived as beautiful. Humans have evolved to experience beauty for the purposes of practical self-benefit, be it procreation, survival, or a promise of pleasure. Evolution has made sure that health is seen is beautiful, because it is health that ensures procreation, pleasure and survival, whereas disease—only kills.

Signs of aging.

Besides the obvious ones, there are tell-tell signs of aging. They manifest themselves in the speed of body movement and speech, in the speed of thinking, of the tissue turnover and speed of growing of skin and hair, and in the body smell. Some people age prematurely: they look and act much older than their age. Their hair and nails grow slowly, their hair is thinned out, no new hairs are growing. Their skin is thick and showing deep wrinkles, as if it the old skin never gets new cell growth. You can see it in their slow body movements, slow speech, reactions, and thinking. They even slouch like someone stereotypically elderly. There is such a thing as a smell of an older person, and some people start smelling like that way before their time. It must be a whole slew of factors that cause it, and pathogens are among them.

People don't generally get more beautiful with age, except during the first two weeks of one's life. All of our lives, we are in a state of slow and constant decomposition into entropy. Just like iron corrodes, our tissues constantly oxidize, the oils in our body grow rancid, our cells produce waste that turns us into a giant dumpster. Life is a constant struggle, and we bare the memories of our battles on our faces, eyes, teeth, skin—everything that reveals the extent of our physical health.

On the other hand, we are in control of ourselves, more that we allow ourselves to believe. We actually can grow old in years, without turning old in the mind and body. There appears to be a definite psychosomatic factor that influences our biological age: we first believe in our youth, then our body adapts to it. I wonder, what would happen to a human who believed that she stopped aging after the age of 15! That would be a curious experiment.

Physical attraction and evolution.

Physical attraction is much less romantic than people would like to believe. It has to do more with survival than anything else. True romantic attraction is all about the mind and soul, and once we realize that, a lot of the pressure to look a certain way will automatically fall off.

What is more important, in my opinion, is tapping into the mechanism of assessing one's health through physical attraction—something that nature designed for us, so we can avoid disease. There are many types of attraction, that often contradict each other.

Opposites attract, because people seek out mates that make up for their perceived deficiencies. The opposite is also true: people who look alike also attract, and it is an incredibly powerful attraction. Looking like a potential mate is a sign of a potential robust union between the two, except the type of similarity is usually not always what everyone expects or perceives.

We already know that people with both very similar and very different DNA to ours are repulsive to us. Yet, I keep seeing these cases, where people with similar or complimentary diseases actually seek each other out. It is as if they are driven by the pathogens inside them to use the human hosts of vehicles to increase their proximity and exchange their DNA for become more evolutionarily robust. The possible mechanism is clear: those pathogens who have manipulated their host to be attracted to others with a chemical environment or a disease that benefits those pathogens,—those pathogens—survive. So, humans should be careful, because not all physical attraction is beneficial to them, some of it may be serving the pathogens they host.

Nutrition.

Besides the cryptic ways that evolution controls our attraction to someone, there are ways that are more accessible to us, and where we can be in control. Nutrition is one of them, and it is a much more powerful beauty tool than mere weight loss. One can be plump, smooth and radiant, and one can be skinny, dried out and shriveled. It is all relative. Physical attractiveness has to do more with the quality of your skin, hair, teeth, and body odor than with your sheer size.

Organic food used to be called just food, before the advent of chemical additives and genetic modifications. That food is the best for our health, and denying that chemicals can do anything to us is like taking poison and denying that it will work. Insanity itself. But we all know that. What's worse is that some organic foods are not very dense with nutrients, because the soil on which they were grown has been long depleted. Foods prepared with fresh and organic ingredients taste mildly sweet and cooling, in contrast to a caustic, metallic, bitter-plastic, heating, or simply tasteless, contaminated foods.

So, traveling to the areas of the world with the richest soils and eating local organic food there—is the only solution that I see. In addition, soils that undergo winter's freeze, have their water restructured, as it is frozen, which adds another value to the food that is grown on it later. Traveling and eating in foreign countries is also beneficial because it lets us ingest their local bacteria, which often carry defense mechanisms for the humans.

Weight loss.

One big glitch in nature is bodily fat deposits. Usually, it works just right, where what's attractive falls within a certain range, somewhere in the middle, that excludes extremely fat and extremely skinny. But modern humans have been so grotesquely infested and overgrown by sugar-seeking bacteria, along with a whole pyramid of pathogens, that they have lost all sense of direction. Now, what would normally be considered sickly thin is considered beautiful, as a reaction to avoid obesity, which does signal poor health and bacteria infestation. However, thin does not mean healthy, either. Cancer makes people thin, as does long-term smoking. Being attracted to thinness is misleading, because it is not directing us to health or any benefit in the survival of the fittest. However, it does testify to our subconscious awareness and attempt to avoid the pathogens that cause obesity.

Adrenal fatigue, caused by exposure to toxic people, to emotional abuse, and to chronic stress of all kinds, also causes inordinate weight gain. In this case, weight sends the right signal of un-attractiveness for a potential mate.

Interestingly enough, social eating is one of the worst things you can do to your body, and it also causes weight gain that rightfully will signal to others one's unattractiveness as a mate. More often than not, social eating excites your body, so that it goes into a low-level fight-or-flight state, interfering with the bile flow and digestion, as well as perceived satiation. Eating on the go has the same effect. I see many people carelessly chewing on a piece of food, with their jaws overly relaxed, their tongue flapping, as they are mechanically smacking away, without tasting the food or properly chewing it.

Finally, uneven weight gain, like swollen stomach, for example, is always a sign of trouble, and so it is rightfully considered unattractive. What I see is that it is caused by the usual suspects: pathogens, adrenal fatigue and lack of vitamins.

There is nothing like sleep.

Sleep is by far the most important factor in preserving one's physical beauty. There is nothing on earth that destroys one's beauty as lack of sleep and lack of rest. Sleep affects every single function in the body, repairing, refreshing and renewing every tissue, and every cell of a human being. Drinking coffee is the worst thing you can do to yourself, especially when you are tired. What you need is sleep, or at least, rest. Coffee not only dehydrates the body, but also blocks adenosine, preventing you from resting when your body needs it most, by blocking the mechanism that makes you tired. It does not actually give you any energy.

Wrinkles and varicose veins.

There are several ideas that I am getting. Chronic coffee drinkers, just like chronic smokers, end up with saggy, prematurely aged skin, depleted of collagen. Orange peel skin can be fixed by eating a lot of hot soups and drinking hot liquids, first thing on an empty stomach. Doing that in the morning is crucial.

The primary cause of crow feet wrinkles (under eyes) is lack of sleep due to worry and being wired up, or any kind of emotional distress. It is not the same as some noise keeping you awake, for example. Skin has two sides: the inner and the outer. The worry wrinkles are form on the inside, and cannot be fixed with any creams or external treatments. Restful sleep is the only cure.

Varicose veins are caused by pathogens. Legs get affected asymmetrically. The patterns of affected areas usually look as if something were climbing up, from the the soles and up toward the heart, like debris being swept up by something—maybe pathogens being swept up by the blood?

Cellulite.

Soon after the economic crisis of 2008, as I remember it now, I suddenly started noticing that virtually every girl in my college town started showing some degree of cellulite. For years afterwards, I have started noticing more and more cellulite on people, as if it was an epidemic. I even noticed it on children, in many countries all over the world—something that I never saw prior.

Of course, all this time, I was doing a lot mental searching for the cause of it, while making all kinds of observations. It became clear to me that cellulite was caused by pathogens, bacterial sugar farming being the main culprit, where the virus causes fat cells grow out of proportion. Interestingly, cellulite shows similar spread patterns to those in varicose veins. Xylitol in an antibacterial that appears to eliminate cellulite. Birch tree juice naturally contains xylitol. So, I did some casual experimenting around. For one person, drinking birch tree juice for a month, a medium size bottle a day, did eliminate all of her cellulite completely! This is not a definitive proof, but only an anecdotal evidence to get people investigating the possibility.

There is some more support for the idea that cellulite is caused by a pathogen, maybe a group of them. In my observations, cellulite goes away with exposure to the sun's UV rays, which do kill bacteria. It also goes away from prolonged swimming in salty water, which is also antibacterial and diuretic.

Edema often accompanies cellulite, and in my modeling, is indicative of inflammation. In fact, swelling and fat often go together, and some people lose a few pounds a day—only by ridding themselves of water,—a known phenomenon. Topical antibacterial substances, like castor and eucalyptus oils, also have an effect on cellulite. The patter is clear to me, and I wish someone would investigate further.

Grey hair and alopecia.

This is another example of pathogens overgrowing in the body, and body's trying to kill them. What? I know, this book is called "Zany Cures", after all. Ok, here is what I see: it is a pathogen trail again. My mind shows me that grey hair is caused by pathogenic overgrowth in the body, and has nothing to do with age, but with pathogen infestation. If only we find what pathogen it is! Or, maybe, we don't have to wait, and can just treat the body with all known antibacterial, antiviral, and anti-fungal agents, and one of them is bound to eliminate this overgrowth.

Many types of alopecia and hair depigmentation are auto-immune diseases, where the infestation of cells happens first, and then the pathogens are attacked by our the immune system. Only when the immune attack happens do people lose hair or hair pigment.

Meats and emotions.

This is something that surprised me! In my visual world, different meats turned out to have different effects on the body, and consequently, on a person's behavior and their attractiveness. Eating chicken makes people energetic and heats up their body. Maybe that is why they recommend eating a chicken soup when one catches a cold. Antibacterial effect, once again! Well, even more heating is duck meat. If you feel sluggish and tired, and cold all over, just eat some duck meat, including fat, and it will give you some energy. Eat that instead of drinking coffee! Fish cools down the body, and calms down agitation. Pork is great for emotional turbulence, it is a great stabilizer. It also can stifle imagination, if eaten in great quantities. Beef makes one feel courageous, and lamb—pacifies the will. Behavior is not exactly phisical, but it affects the physique and physical attractiveness of a person. Once again, I am only reporting what I am seeing in my ideasthetic mind.

Of course, I tried all these remedies on myself, and they actually all worked.

Body odor.

Some people smell like metal: this is a particular rancid smell that you can also smell when oils get old, in expired beauty products and in old food. For example, everybody has smelled that old fish smell that is just unbearable. The people smell this way because they are oxidizing, they are overwhelmed with free radicals and pathogenic infestations, and it is a sign of a pre-cancer state. Some people smell nauseatingly sweet, and that is just sugar, fermenting in their cells, a sign that they are under attack from gold-mining bacteria, and other pathogens will be arriving soon. I noticed that diabetic children smell like that, in particular. The only solution I see is getting rid of bacterial overgrowth, and the remedies are plentiful.

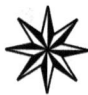

CONCLUSION

So as not to end the book on unpleasant body odor, and leave a lasting aftertaste of stench in the mouth of the reader, let's talk about something positive—an equivalent of sniffing coffee beans!

The main idea that permeates every single line in this book is that we are in control of our bodies, that we don't have to get old and be unattractive simply because we are older. What I have seen in my mind—is phantasmagorical, yet it seems to make sense. It just does not have any proof, yet. I do hope that medical professionals will consider pathogenic causes for the currently incurable diseases. And I do hope that everyone will dare to see old age and death itself curable, even if temporarily.

If any of my ideasthetic visualizations can ever lead to finding one single effective, standardized, and replicable cure to save a single life—then, zany is good, and I haven't lived or written in vain.

www.ingramcontent.com/pod-product-compliance
Lightning Source LLC
Chambersburg PA
CBHW071031280326
41935CB00011B/1531